The Snow Globe Journals

....sound bites from a mental illness

Suzy Johnston

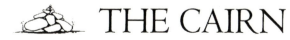
THE CAIRN

Published by
The Cairn,
Brincliffe,
West Dhuhill Drive,
Helensburgh G84 9AW

www.thecairn.com

A catalogue record of this book is available from the British Library.

ISBN 978 0 9548092 2 5

I am indebted to the following for their help and assistance:

Clunie Group Ltd, Oban. www.cg-ltd.co.uk – *formatting*
Brian Averall, The Lennox Herald – *portrait*
Pixart Pictures, Helensburgh – *front cover design*

Acknowledgements and Thanks

A HUGE thank you to my family and the friends who continue to bewilder me with their love and support – especially Pat Pollok-Morris and Polly Dunlop.

To the many consultants along with the medical staff and nursing teams of both the Acute Medical Ward 6 and the Christie Ward (psychiatry) at the Vale of Leven Hospital who were involved in treating me when I became so seriously ill last year - my eternal thanks and appreciation for their life-saving care of both my physical and mental health throughout 2008 and their unending compassion, patience and good humour. Also to my pharmacists at Boots The Chemist, Helensburgh sincere thanks for their professional expertise, interest and kindness. A massive thank you to each and every one of the doctors, nurses and receptionists at Dr Calder's Practice in Helensburgh – especially Dr Liz Underwood for her wisdom, concern, insight, empathy and patience. I guess we all have our own battles to fight – well, Dr Underwood you certainly made mine a hell of a lot easier.

Sincere thanks to Dr Raj Persaud for his kind words at the beginning of this book and finally a BIG thank to DM, my unswerving and truly fantastic CPN who speaks so much sense it's frightening!

And to anyone who reads this book? Take a deep breath, keep on living your life and don't give up – there is so much more to still come.

Suzy Johnston,
January 2009

Helplines – UK and Ireland

www.aware.ie –1890 303 302

www.breathingspacescotland.co.uk – 0800 83 85 87 (Scotland only)

Careline – 020 8514 1177

www.nhs24.com – 0845 424 24 24

www.samaritans.org.uk – 08457 90 90 90

www.sane.org.uk – 0845 767 8000

For other countries – call your emergency health service number and ask for details of mental health support numbers or agencies.

Mental Health Websites

www.carers.org

www.chooselife.net

www.mdf.org.uk

www.mind.org.uk

www.mentalhealth.org.uk

www.nami.org

www.pendulum.org.

www.penumbra.org.uk

www.rethink.org

www.rcpsych.ac.uk

www.ru-ok.com   adolescent website

www.samh.org.uk

www.scottishrecovery.net

www.seemescotland.org.uk

www.shift.org.uk

www.slam.nhs.uk

Music and lyrics on surviving mental illness and self-harm

www.badalicemusic.com – cd – download ***Walk in my Shoes***

Dedications

This book is dedicated to Michel.

What can I say? You are my umbrella when the skies open, you are the drink that slakes my thirst and after all that? You simply take hold of my hand. I love you for now and forever............and that's a mighty long time.

Suzy x

In memory of

Laurence Wilson

Chair, Bipolar Fellowship Scotland 2003-2008

CONTENTS

Preface

In this her second book on living with mental illness, Suzy Johnston takes the reader of *'The Snow Globe Journals'* further into the realms of that feared unknown – the dark and murky world of psychosis. The clarity of her experiences gives a remarkably revealing insight into what the psychotic experience is like with its frightening lack of control of thoughts and its total detachment from reality. She illustrates powerfully and articulates vividly the inability of an intelligent mind to differentiate between the real world and the psychotic one.

It was in her autobiography *'The Naked Bird Watcher'* – an optimistic account on managing a mental illness - that Suzy gave a revealing, comprehensive insight into her world of mental distress, its challenges and symptoms along with the pivotal role of recovery and its management. Having established an international reputation as a respected writer and voice within the mental health movement, she became columnist for the 'This Life' column for Mental Health Today Magazine, a contributor to leading journals such as the British Medical Journal on living with her condition along with writing articles for newspapers both in the UK and abroad. When her mother Jean Johnston wrote *'To Walk on Eggshells'* their books emerged as the first joint publications from both a patient and the carer on living with a mental illness and managing its recovery. Suzy's partner, Michel Syrett, has joined the daughter and mother duo in giving talks and presentations throughout the UK on mental illness issues, stigma, recovery and the role of the carer. They are frequent guests on programmes relating to mental health topics. As The Cairn Team they offer training, education and awareness presentations on all mental illness issues, recovery and the role of the carer and can be contacted via The Cairn website – **www.thecairn.com**

The BBC Radio documentary *'Being Suzy Johnston'* was short listed in the Mental Health Media Awards. Determined to normalize mental illness, Suzy's ability to raise awareness and normalise mental illness was recognised by the Girl Guide Movement who included her in their list of 100 Inspirational Women. She is also a musician/song writer and recorded *Walk in my Shoes* with Bad Alice which is available from **www.badalicemusic.com**. Its lyrics are based on surviving mental illness, self-harm and the issues that face the young of today. Suzy and Michel have their home in the West coast of Scotland.

The Naked Bird Watcher *by Suzy Johnston,*
ISBN 0954809203

To Walk on Eggshells *by Jean Johnston,*
ISBN 0954809211

www.thecairn.com

www.badalicemusic.com

Foreword

Psychosis is an experience of endless fascination to both scientists, who are attempting to understand it, doctors who must treat it, patients who endure and sometimes revel in it, and the lay public who frequently fear it.

Suzy Johnston has accomplished an audacious and rare undertaking in penning an unusually frank account of a psychotic breakdown. If that was all that she had done the book would still be worth reading – but something much more important is being undertaken here.

Despite all the research effort that has been invested all over the world, the medical model still struggles to capture the psychotic experience. Questionnaires, interview schedules, blood tests and brain scanners have all been deployed in an attempt to illuminate what is going on in psychosis, and although meaningful leaps have been and continue to be made in our understanding, it's still the case that we probably know least about the psychotic mind, compared to all other experiences that fall within the medical remit.

Perhaps one key piece in the jigsaw that has been missing is the detailed first person account – and it's easy to see why this has been problematic in incorporating these into the scientific view. Once people recover from psychosis, it is not a part of their lives they necessarily relish revisiting, indeed their memory for it seems to fade rapidly, a bit like a vivid dream after one has awakened in the morning from a feverish sleep.

But the extended first person account is something I believe psychiatry ignores at its peril for I contend it's only a blow by blow description over an extended period which holds out any hope of illuminating what it's really like to undergo some of the most frightening and vivid experiences open to humankind.

We have too easily jumped to conclusions in modern psychiatry that we know what someone is going through when, for example, they answer yes to the typical hasty screening question asked distractedly in the Casualty Department - 'Do you hear voices?'

In fact not only is there a vast individual variability we neglect to our peril, but trying to get at what its really like to have these experiences can only be properly elucidated by detailed and coherent first person accounts like the one you currently hold in your hands. While brain scanning and blood tests have their place, they are never going to tell us what it feels like when the brain and mind stray beyond the limits of experience that you can discuss meaningfully with your neighbour.

In my clinical experience treating psychosis on a daily basis at The Bethlem Royal and Maudsley NHS Hospitals Trust, part of the complexity of the issue is the unique sense of isolation enduring a psychotic breakdown engenders.

Clinicans like myself are not just wrestling with the convolution of an intricate mechanism like the mind appearing to not function in an understandable manner, but each person reacts differently to their psychotic experience – and each person's family, friends and neighbours seem to do so as well.

It's only when the wider public and policy makers come to understand how dreadfully difficult managing psychosis and assisting sufferers is, that proper resources might at last begin to be diverted to properly treating this serious and common medical emergency.

This, and for a whole host of other reasons, is why this book is so very important.

Raj Persaud FRCPsych
'The Mind'

The Snow Globe Journals

By Suzy Johnston

INTRODUCTION

Sometimes, when I am alone, I open my mouth and sing as loudly as I can. No particular tune is required (and I'm not a great singer). No, I'm just embracing the joy of being alive and revelling in the fact that at one time I came so close to the edge that I needed a multitude of helping hands to keep me from falling.

This book explores those dark times in grave detail and goes far deeper and closer to the bone than my previous book, "The Naked Bird Watcher". I needed to do this because I felt I had formerly shied away from those thoughts and emotions, partly because I wasn't yet ready to fully address them and also because I truly wondered whether anyone would be interested in reading about them. I guess I'll find out the answer to that one!

In this book I've split the text into three sections: illness/hospital/the journey home. In the first section, I've used every literary technique I could think of to express the trauma that I was going through at that time – metaphors, analogies, descriptive text, bad grammar – and experimented with text size to increase impact.

In the second section, I wanted to give a more well-rounded feel to what it means to be a patient in a 21st Century psychiatric ward. Again, I have to acknowledge that I am extremely fortunate in that my local psychiatric ward (The Christie Ward) is a truly excellent facility and I was always treated with compassion, kindness, respect and care.

The third section is all about that buzz word of today – recovery. I believe it is hugely important to point out here that whilst I feel as though I have "recovered" I am not CURED. Recovery and cure are two very different terms and whilst I am functioning well and no longer need to be in hospital, I am still bothered by suicidal thoughts, depression, paranoia and occasional delusions. This, I have had to accept, is all a part of being me. So I will continue to live my life, realise how lucky I have been and hopefully pass on a few thoughts and ideas that will help others in the same boat to fight off the monsters that continue to haunt them.

Take care.
S x

Part 1 : Illness

I am a snow globe. There are times when my head and thoughts are so clear and pure that I feel as though some small fragment of God is flowing through my flawed arteries. Is that blasphemous? Surely in this 21st Century reality show that we live in, we have left blasphemy WAY behind? Whatever. Do you care?

Then someone, something picks me up and shakes me. I am a maelstrom of tiny stars, lunar fragments and space dust. I lose all perspective. I...Can't.... Think. Keep shaking you son of a bitch, keep shaking. Because I know where this will end.....like everything else......in confusion and darkness.

Maybe, if you could put your coffee cup down for a second, you could come and bear witness. And hey! Bring the family! I puke regret and shame. And I kid myself that the pills will cure me. Will they? Won't they? What is my future?

I am just a snow globe.

And I break when I fall.

A Beginning (of sorts)

Does your conscience whisper to you in the dead of night…. and do you think about killing yourself so much so that there isn't room for anything else? Will you listen or do you roll over in the apparent safety of your bed eager to escape the edgy whispers that surround you? When does worry become paranoia? When do doubts become delusions? Where ultimately is that thin, shaky, pencil grey line between sanity and insanity?

You're going to judge me by what you read on these flimsy will o' the wisp pieces of paper. That's okay. Don't worry about it – I'd do the same, anyone would. So, exactly why am I writing this stuttering prose, this stream of consciousness anyway? Hmm. Because I want to? Yes. Because I NEED to? Even more so. What I crave most of all is simple: catharsis – a way of quieting and extricating the ringing in my brain, the fire alarm screaming in my head and the finger nails scraping down the inside of my skull. This is the labour and the trial that I have chosen…..or maybe it chose me. I WILL be true to myself and if that shocks or offends? So be it.

But there's some merit in this, and not self serving merit at that. I believe, honestly, that an arduous life is still a life worth living. Of that I have no doubt. Even amidst all this darkness there is still hope and light – things that make you smile and give you the determination to carry on.

Inside. That's where the light eventually comes from you

know. Pretty clichéd isn't it? But it's irrevocably true. Okay, so some believe "the light" is God or Buddha or something but let's face it – you can have every God in history batting in your corner but unless you believe in YOURSELF you ain't going anywhere. Maybe you need medication and maybe not. I do. Maybe you need counselling. I need that too. These tools give you the ability to push your way through the darkness with the light beaming out of you. Don't ever quit. Because even if the light seems to falter and fade it hasn't really gone. You've just momentarily closed your eyes, that's all. Open them again. Be bold and open them again and see your future spanning out in front of you.

PSYCHOSISandthisiswhatitislike…

(An experience of psychosis)

Psychosis lurks and any thoughts of control are NOT POSSIBLE. Insight is a faraway dream that flits away like an Autumn leaf in the wind. This is how I know Hell to be.

Evil thoughts spiral out of me in an uncontrollable abandonment of all I ever intended or wanted to be in this World. I am nauseous and dirt fills my hollow bones. I cannot hear, see, smell, touch, or feel in any coherent fashion. I am lost, lost, lost and damned for all eternity. Nothing makes sense. I can't focus – too much of everything, too little of nothing. A SCREAM, a shout, something hurting. Was that me? Was that today? What the fuck is going on? HELP. Interference rains down from infernal satellites above clogging up my brain and rendering me hopeless and exhausted. My skin is tarnished and grey and only my duvet offers comfort and the chance to hide. There is no light today, I learn. My mantra burns: "This too shall pass. This too shall pass." I hold onto it with the determination of a newborn clinging to its mother's breast. "This too shall pass. This too shall pass."

My eyes and ears are open - but depression and psychosis cast a film over them that is opaque and consuming and dangerous. Everything is contaminated in this World today. Time shows no sympathy and stretches each second like an impossible elastic band for a hysterical eon.

How we laugh. Like lepers.

Tissue Paper Seatbelt
(Escaping the demons)

Am I a bungee jumper with a faulty cord who should just philosophically accept my fate? No, I'm stubborn like that. Just ask my friends.

So how do I extricate myself from such a seemingly impossible situation? Hmm. Is the glass half empty or half full? Frankly, who cares if the glass is even there – I had to find my way out or all that crap would have taken me down. There are many rungs on life's ladder but at the bottom there is always the abyss waiting, lurking, calling out in the darkness. Don't ever look down. What do I do? Well first I panic. Of course I do, I'm human! Then, and this takes an articulated truck's worth of strength, I say something out loud. I do this for two reasons: 1. To distract me from the constant noise in my head. 2. To help me get used to how it sounds before I make my next step – CALL SOMEONE.

Calling someone is nowhere as easy as it sounds. Oh no. First of all I convince myself that, like a tissue paper seatbelt, I am a colossal waste of time and that no one in anything approaching their right mind would give even the tiniest piece of excrement about me. Second, I'm certain that everyone hates me anyway and thirdly I believe that absolutely NOTHING anyone has to say will make the slightest bit of difference because what the hell do they know about what's going on in my head???

You know what? THIS IS THE ILLNESS TALKING AND YOU HAVE TO GET ROUND IT. So I pick up the phone and call whoever I can. I forget what time it is and forget about what I expect to hear at the end of the line. If you are in need of help don't quit until you get that help. It's true that in times of crisis you truly find out who's in your corner. I wish with all my heart that this wasn't the case. It's a bruising road – there's no getting away from that.

So. I've looked at one way to help yourself out of a potentially dangerous situation: calling someone – well, there's more you can do. What exactly? Basically I do ANYTHING that helps distract me from those murderous thoughts (although loading up on booze and/or drugs will only make you self destruct further. Besides as alcohol's a depressant and drugs screw up your brain it doesn't take a genius to figure out what effect they'll have on your already precarious state of mind.) So. I listen to music. I eat and smell an orange. I watch TV. I jump up and down for God's sake, ANYTHING to inject something different and positive into the status quo. I play my guitar or talk to my cat. Both help. This isn't rocket science. I find out what works for me, and yes, something WILL work (don't give up). And oh yeah, so what if it makes me look a little foolish or undignified! This is saving my life that I'm talking about here so dignity can take a good long running jump!

Next step? Removing myself (literally) from the situation. It doesn't matter how rotten I feel, and believe me there's been times where my whole body feels like it is stuck in some leech infested molasses. I HAVE to get up, force myself to move and get myself to a different, SAFER location.

For a kick off if I'm in the bedroom I go into the sitting room and put the TV on. You get the idea. Then I call someone and get them to come over. I find it's best to call their mobile (if they have one) so that they can stay on the line as they get to my place. If someone's in the house I WAKE THEM UP. I don't let myself think "Damn, they'll be pissed off..." that doesn't matter – can you imagine how they'd feel if I didn't wake them up and something happened?

When the suicidal thoughts leer at me and consume my thoughts, I'm not in a rational state of mind so it's crucial that I surround myself with as many RATIONAL people as possible. Why? So that they can help me break down the muddy walls of irrationality which tower high around me and give me the reason and clarity that I need in order to make it through this sharkinfestedjunglemare that sneeringly dances in my head. I promise you that there is always a way out of this, no matter how unlikely it seems.

Purgatory

(The motivation to keep going)

Sometimes I hate myself. It's true, I do.   It's just the way I feel about myself , so deal with it. I do. I hate myself because everyday I have to cautiously test out my brain before I gingerly let my senses take over, before I even exhale, to see whether this is another day I can struggle through or whether this is IT – the day I finally kill myself and cause untold pain to those who love me. Self, self, self. I am unwanted yet I am needed. Everything depends on thinking about the source: myself. I must concentrate on every nuance, every second and every breath. Dying must not become my life. But I am far from perfect and slip, slide my way to the 64 million dollar question which of course is "Why, if I claim to hate myself so much, am I not dead yet?" I can think of a hundred reasons why I should be. But before I get all self indulgent and dramatic let me give you the honest answer: friends, family, the medical profession who give me such great support, hell, even the woman who chats to me as she sells me my newspaper in the morning – all of these people give me a purpose, a drive to keep going. I might want to mess with my life, but I certainly DON'T want to mess with theirs. So I will carry on breathing in and out enjoying this air of ours that, on the surface, seems so pure but at its heart is dark and polluted. Kind of like me if you get my drift.

Suicide

Suicide is NEVER the solution and I believe this to be true. Really. It removes any ability I might have had to solve whatever terrors I was dealing with. THEY WIN. Get it? THEY WIN. Plus of course, I'm leaving everyone whoever cared about me a huge vat of pain, grief and maybe-I-could-have-stopped-her guilt to wallow in. That's a pretty shitty thing to do.

Is suicide or attempted suicide a sin? Personally I don't think trying to kill yourself is a rational act and is therefore beyond moral judgement. What do you think? Frankly though, does anyone HONESTLY think it would be of benefit to condemn a failed suicide as a sinner??? Surely that person has enough going on without that to deal with as well? The same goes for a family bereaved by suicide.

I KNOW it can be frustrating, that suicide can seem like the only way out – the only way to silence the vitriolic chaos in your head – in fact often it's NOT that people actually want to kill themselves it's just that they are so desperate for the pain and torment to STOP that as a consequence they find themselves falling through the irreturnable void. But this is YOUR life. Don't throw it away no matter how tormented it has become. There is always another way out and people on hand to help you. I know how it feels to be walking through a tunnel that is caving in on all sides but even in that tunnel there is hope and something, no matter how small, to live for. Think about your dog, the fresh Spring leaves on the trees, your brother, your best friend, watching your football team next season. All these things await you and offer you a future.

Private

(Intimacy difficulties when you're mentally unwell)

Intimacy has been slowly suffocated in a dusty drawer to which I have the only key. It has been hidden in a place long forgotten (on purpose of course). Entry is UTTERLY forbidden to everyone.

Even you.

And especially me.

Creeping Dirt

(Feelings of self loathing)

I can't get clean. No matter how much I shower, bathe, exfoliate, scrub, scrape and rub the oily film of stinking, putrid dirt that coats my skin remains resolute.

Soap, shampoo, conditioner, body lotion, face scrub, coco-fucking-nut shell skin purifier for God's sake! All use-less. Under my nails is the worst. It makes me nervous. I will strip my skin and leave my bones pristine and shining .....but....but what if the contamination goes deeper? Now I can feel the rank swirl pumping through my blackened arteries, clogging my veins and bunging up my feeble excuse for a heart like snot from a three week old cold that just isn't shifting.

This sickness desolates me. I am rotting from within, soiled and loathsome – if only you could see it. How you would leave.

"You're a nuisance. And I don't like dirt."

The Breeders

Careless lives

Ever found yourself crossing a road without checking the traffic? Taken one, two, three too many pills? Or quietly sat locked in the toilet with a razor blade thinking "What if?" before silently putting it away and returning to watch TV with your family. These are dangerous paths littered with the winsome, careless remain of victims and truants. Two words shine out in the murky depths of the bog and the mire: find help, little one.....FIND HELP.

Endless

I'm just coping with coping. Scrabbling my way through each day and each day and each day and on and on in an endless scratching void. Breathe in? My lungs rattle, bitch and moan and my body spits the life giving air out vehemently and with disgust. Breathe out? The vacuum that is now my body threatens to suck the skin off my bones. AND I WANT TO SCREAM!!!!!!!!

The Road

(Facing mental illness – trying to cross to safety)

The road leers at me. It's tarmaced hard as fuck and oh man this'll hurt if you fall down surface smells of dirt and ghosts – ghosts that roar by in shiny, windowed capsules that paint my world with coughing fits and pollution. They don't care. Not really. They're too fast to die. Too fast to be bothered with the likes of stupid, doubting me.

I want to step out off the relative safety of the pavement because the other side beckons clear and pure, but I'm scared. Not of death but of forever being lost in the Styx like river of traffic that has opened up in front of me. I swear a mist has fallen. What time is it? How long have I been standing here? It doesn't matter. It's not as though I really exist anyway....

(Too Contrived)

(A tightly wound ball of contradictions)

I'm too much. Too little. Too bold. Too scared and wary. Too concrete. Too fragile. Too unhappy. Too ecstatic. Too gentle. Too insensitive. Too brave. Too frightened. Too real. Too fake. Too pure. Too contaminated. Too lost. Too found. Too victorious. Too much of a fucking loser. Too proud. Too uncertain. Too confident. Too unsure. Too certain. Too mixed up. Too bruised. Too healed. To much me. Too little everyone else. Too sorted. Too up shit creek. Too dumb. Too smart. Too simple. Too complex....Too contradictory.

An eyelash in a storm.

A cat in the rain.

A flower in the dark.

Let me change places please.

Let me change.

Self Harm

"How do you feel when you can't feel?
How do you fly when there's no sun?
How do see through all those tears?
How do you know when you're not the only one?"

Bad Alice

Cut...Slice...Carve...Hack...Chop...Attack.

Cut...Slice...Carve...Hack...Chop...Attack

However I chose to describe it to myself I had to deal with the fact that ultimately self harm is just a means (and a crude one at that) and not the "end" - the solution – that I was desperately searching for. Who the Hell was I kidding??? I didn't have a clue what I was doing. All I knew was that the screaming...SCREAMING, FLAILING NUMBNESS in my dissolving brain was crying out for something, ANYTHING, to distract it from the inwardly crumbling cartoon shell that used to be me. I pretend I'm winning: that every "holy shit what if someone sees it!" scar is some sort of pathetic notch on my survival bed post. Razors and elastoplast. Two sides of a marked coin. One to open, one to hide. One to fake a private victory, one to cover a public embarrassment. And the power I wield? Withered and empty, kidding myself over and over again. There is no pain, no physical pain anyway; like that matters. I just want to FEEL. Something, anything, whatever, however. Just something I can put my finger on and say

"Hey, that's REAL" instead of this numbing, voidless, soundless, bastard NOTHING that lazily and sickeningly rotates around my head like the most messed up Merry-Go-Round in the world.

So what am I left with? Parallel lines on my arms – tracks to Desperateville and tattoos of pointless angst. I did it because nothing else short of killing myself offered anything even CLOSE to a way out – a momentary respite. Hell, all I was looking for was a damn break for a few seconds! I need to get back in touch with who I was, or, more accurately, who I needed to be in order to survive this life which I had arrived in outwardly screaming and had now internalised and become consumed by that self same expression.

I cut quite far up my arms so that my friends wouldn't accidentally see – although once I had to do some quick explaining/lying with a face as red as the blood that I had smudged on my skin only a few hours earlier. Being caught wasn't an option. This wasn't some attention seeking "Check me out, I'm so angst ridden and cool I cut myself". This wasn't some fucking fashion statement – if you think that you're missing the point. The bell jar that surrounded me just wasn't shifting and try as I might I couldn't hear, see, taste, smell or feel anything through the thick, opaque glass. Are you beginning to understand why the sharpness of a razor cut and the life affirming validation of seeing, touching and, yes, even tasting my own blood gave me? And you know what? It was fucking STUPID. I see that now.

I have spoken to quite a few people about self harm and whilst EVERYONE is keen to know "Why?" or "What did you do?" or even "what did it FEEL like?", NO ONE EVER ASKED ME "WHY DID YOU STOP?" which, let's face it, is the most important question of all.

I stopped for two reasons:

1. I was becoming more and more frightened at my increasing loss of control and the spiralling increase in frequency of my self harming. This wasn't what I had ever intended to become but self harm CAN be addictive and once this path is chosen it can be bloody difficult to reroute and save yourself.

2. I was becoming increasingly sure that my friends were becoming suspicious about my destructive antics. In some ways I resented and felt angry at my friends for this. My friends! This was my business and I wanted NO external interference thank-you-very-much not from friends, family, my boyfriend, doctors or psychiatrists – they could all keep their beaks out of it. But in reality? In the most frightened corner of my heart I knew I needed them all now more than ever. I needed their help if I was going to get out of this. Ever noticed how much easier it is to slide down a shute in a kid's playground than climb up it? That's what this was like. So I dragged myself, slipping and sliding up that damned slide until finally, FINALLY I reached the safety and security of the top. You know what I realised when I got there? One, the view was marvellous. Two, I didn't have to feel ashamed anymore or dirty or guilty or angry or any of those pent up negative emotions that had actually been CAUSED by self harm – my "solution" – and not banished by it like I had originally planned and meticulously theorized.

Okay, so those are the "Whys", now for the "Hows". I hit things. Soft things like pillows, cushions and my mattress. I cranked up my stereo and yelled like a dervish. I thrashed at my electric guitar in a full volume frenzy of hatred, desperation and revulsion until the numbing pain which had consumed and controlled me began.....began to lose its grip on my scarred being as I began to exorcise it from my brain in a stuttering, those shoes don't fit anymore, progression. Surviving self harming and coming out of the other side aren't things you're encouraged to put on your CV but I regard them as two of my finest personal triumphs. I can feel now in a healthy way and when that coma like asphyxiation and dull ache return, and they do at times, it's not the razor I reach for anymore but the phone to call a friend or book an appointment with my GP or psychiatrist. I had to learn the hard way, that to deal with those thoughts on my own left me all too vulnerable to negative coping strategies. I can't afford to let myself be in that place again. Ever.

"Sweet and divine, razor blade shine
Day after day, cutting away,
Day after day, but anyway....."

Foo Fighters

Can someone explain......?

Sometimes I wonder just what the hell I am doing here? I feel like a piece of a discarded jigsaw which doesn't quite fit regardless of the impatient hammerings of the petulant thumb that won't take no for an answer.

I don't think I am alone. Why do I live in this town? Why do I wear these clothes? Are these people really my friends? And if so, why? Why do I like apples but hate apple juice? And why does ANYONE eat sweetcorn???

I'm baffled by life's simplicities and mystified by its solutions......WHAT ON EARTH IS GOING ON??????

Don't Look Too Closely...

Have you ever had anyone tell you that you are seeing or hearing things that aren't there? HOW THE HELL DO THEY KNOW ANYWAY???

I see giant insects. I wish I didn't but I do. My heart struggles to beat constricted by the icy sweat that is freezing HARD around it. I'm caught in the headlights of an oncoming HGV that's rumbling contentedly along at 70mph and ain't stopping for no one, no sir. I'm terrified. But? Well, but even fear, even TERROR loses its edge after a while and gradually I find my heart begins to break free of its icy cage and stubbornly refuse to be scared and intimidated by things I see. With mental superglue I stick the fragments of my nerves and sanity back together, carefully blocking out the darkness that greedily creeps between. I play a game of poker and, as time passes and experience grows, my hand gets stronger but, oh, it's how you play those cards!

Yes, I am scared but I have learned that this too shall pass. Fear is not in itself something to really be afraid of. Really.

Embarrassment....
and laughter on all sides

A moment to ponder.......so far this book has been all about mental illness but here I want to highlight the very real fact that we all possess mental health and are capable of enjoying life and having a laugh even when diagnosed with a psychiatric disorder. The reason I feel it is important to highlight this is two fold: 1. Mental illness is not always a constant feature in your life and for me there are times of respite where life is very much for living and 2. this is the story of MY life and it would be an unfair representation to only mention the negative side – funny things happen to me too y'know and I thought I'd share one with you.......

My younger brother, Ollie, and I were standing languidly in a "they're all the same anyway coffee bar" trying to order iced coffees, sorry, frappachinos (note to self: ordering coffee is the REAL reason for further education as the complexity of this seemingly MINDLESS task is ridiculous!) Anyway, Ollie and I had just ordered – a combination of relief at getting the bloody task over with and irritated annoyance at the smug beautiful people who seem to live/breathe/work/breed in these places and manage to trip the words grande-americano-skinny-caramel-latte-with chocolate sprinkles off their tongues as though:

a) they have some sort of deeper, hidden meaning and

b) with absolutely no trace of shame WHATSOEVER that they sound like complete McConsumer urbanite unit shifters

The nice but cloned girl serving us (pretty, bright and bored to death) commented idly that she liked my necklace and where did it come from? When I replied that I didn't actually know as it was a gift from my boyfriend she turned to the unsuspecting Ollie and said "So where did you get it?"

At this point Ollie's head exploded or at least that's what he wished to have had happened as, no doubt, to any young man the embarrassment of being taken for your older sister's boyfriend is almost preferable to being crucified by your testicles. Well, marginally.

The poor girl was distracted from punching our bill out as she was equally mortified at her error and you could just tell that she was quietly and resignedly waiting for the inevitable insertion of her other foot into her mouth. Sure enough......"You just look so close" she stuttered. "No...I mean...not in that way...oh God!"

Time to save the day, I felt, and reassured "Wishing to God She Had Never Opened Her Mouth In The First Place" that if I found out from my boyfriend where he got the necklace I'd come into the shop and tell her. Then I kissed Ollie on the cheek, called him "Darling", grabbed our frappathingies and dragged him shrieking out of the shop.

Postscript: Ollie and I made it out onto the street, stopped and looked at each other in silence.....and then howled with laughter! Ain't brothers grand!!!

Countdown

16 minutes and 42 seconds. The car drove on at a speed mocking the 35mph on the dashboards lazy speedometer. I wanted to be sick. 16 minutes and 31 seconds. Trees rushed past our stationary car laughing and commenting on my shaky disposition and nervous eyes. Confusion and panic weighed heavy on me. My heart raced although with what I was unclear. 16 minutes and 23 seconds. In the front Mum and Kit chatted with easy confidence and careless abandon. Internally I SCREAMED. 16 minutes and 9 seconds. Keep it together. Smoke another cigarette. Fuck, nearly out. Must get more. 20, 40 today? Who cares, not me. This journey has been torture – at least 2 miles of sitting still clutching my lifelines: cigarettes and....and.... check watch, shit, 15 minutes and 56 seconds until I can take my next pill; the 5mm diameter yellow pill that is pretty much the only thing that is stopping me from ripping out my jugular with my bare hands at the moment. 15minutes and 44 seconds. Time ticks ever backwards. I dig my nails into my legs as a form of distraction. Tick, tick, tick. Help me someone. 15 minutes and 37 seconds. My watch is nearly worn out from my continual sweaty gaze. Tick, tick, tick. 15 minutes and 31 seconds. I think I'm going to die. 15 minutes and 27 seconds.

"STAY AWAY!"

Nirvana

Part 2 : Hospital

13

(First day on readmission to the Ward)

Thirteen. No. Can't go there. Forbidden. Taboo. Unclean. A shaking agitated finger waved at me from underneath the protective curtain of the opposite bed. Bed 11. I had just arrived in the ward and was full to bursting with depression, psychosis and paranoia. I really didn't need this disembodied finger pointing at me and invisible but aggressive voice forbidding me to put my heavier by the second suitcase down beside Bed 13.

"Leave me alone." Begged once, twice, three times for vocalisation swiftly followed by a bolder but much less likely "Stay the fuck away from me!"

However, before I could as far as open my mouth I gave an involuntary shudder as the perpetrator from the increasingly frightening territory on the other side of the room crawled out from under the jollily patterned curtain which fell like a Satanic cape on her shoulders. Even before she rose to her feet she shrieked in a voice hinting at confusion and fear "You can't have that Bed; it's number 13!!!" and then, rather dramatically, "IT'S CURSED!!!"

Had I been feeling better I think I would have pointed out that the only bad luck that Bed 13 had brought me was this rather surreal entrance to the ward which frankly I was having a bit of trouble getting my own messed up head around! As it was I was just too freaked out to respond so I just stood there, holding my suitcase and waited for something else to happen. I didn't have to wait long – in the following 10 seconds two nurses came in, one to escort my obviously distressed neighbour back to the comparative safety and superstition free zone of Bed 11 and one to reassure me that IT WAS ALL GOING TO BE JUST FINE (I think the capital letters were for my benefit!)

The List

As it turned out Bed 13 was to be my crucifix for the next three months – the place where I begged , cried and prayed for redemption, suffered the cruel yet tantalizing agony of recovery and eventually glimpsed that brightest of visions, salvation.

By the time my tensed, screwed up body hit the mattress for the first time I hadn't slept in 3 months and was deathly certain about five, in my mind, irrefuetable facts:

1. I was THE most evil person on the planet.

2. The nurses and doctors were plotting to kill me.

3. I was not ill. There was NOTHING wrong with me.

4. My parents were planning to evict me and when they succeeded I would have to live penniless in London for the remainder of my life.

5. I HAD, above all else, to kill myself.

"I'd like to help you doctor
Yes I really, really would
But the din in my head is too much
And it's no good"

Suzanne Vega

Twenty a day

By the second day I had somewhat shakily organised a cig-arette regime for myself in which my twenty a day cigarette allowance was very carefully spread throughout the day. There were no 'spares' for emergencies – I simply didn't have the resources so there had to be NO mistakes. God, even the IDEA that I might run out sent me into mental spasms and contortions.

Smoking a cigarette involved ritual and routine and both of these helped keep me semi sane. As such each cigarette was a crucial focus that I desperately needed in a world that seemed to be spinning in a somewhat lurching fashion ever closer to the wretched precipice of "buggered-if-I-want-to-look-down-thank-you-sunshine".

Smoking a cigarette, at my pace, and if the thoughts didn't interrupt and leave me frozen in my chair with silvery ash burnt down to my nicotine stained fingers, took around 4½ minutes. If I made myself walk slowly down the corridor, through reception and on up to the smoke room (where I would carefully select as isolated a chair as possible) and then afterwards again force myself to pad slowly back the whole process could take up to 5½ minutes. That was 5½ minutes of not having to think about killing myself or all of that other crazy shit that was bouncing around in my skull. THAT'S how important smoking was to me. And why.

Of course, the social risks involved with smoking were

HUGE. For a kick off you could only smoke in the commandingly named "Smoke Room " but that meant mixing with people and I found the whole concept that someone might ask me for 'a light' or, even worse, actually sit down beside me and try to converse TERRIFYING. Believe me, at that point in my life, I was having so much trouble of making sense of what was going on in MY head without trying to understand someone else's thoughts or comments on life. So, I gawped fixedly at the murky TV screen just praying to Christ that everyone would please leave me alone. Mercifully they did, until gradually and with a creaking grace I began to let people back into my grainy world.

Clocks

(When I was first admitted the Ward was brand new and the clocks had not yet been put up on the walls).

Ten past ten. The ward clock smiled benevolently down on me taking pity on my furrowed brow and wrapped-in-gorse-stay-away-tensed-body. When I had entered the confines of the ward three days (I think?) earlier there had been no time only meals, medication and silently prowling nurses be-decked in soft soled shoes which reeked of stealth and efficiency.

I recall darkness – night I suppose, but still my psyche ached for time. I had no watch and the entire place, brand new as it was, was absent of clocks.

How long had I been lying here staring aimlessly out of the window? Two minutes? Two hours? Two months??? When, if, maybe, was someone coming to visit? Had I slept or just slipped into a waking dream of incomprehensible length? Was I early? Was I late? When had this begun and more importantly how would I know when it had finished?

And then the men in cornflower blue overalls appeared with clocks for EVERYONE – or every room at least – but left them, left them, LEFT THEM all set at ten past ten. They stayed in their fixed grin for two days and then, after a gentle nudge by the cornflower blue brigade, began to go about the very proper business of telling the time.

I needed time desperately. I needed its certainty and point of reference. But, and it was a big but, how I missed the comforting, optimistic reflections of a clock that in its stasis reminded me of what the future could hold for me once again.

not quite dead......

I swear to you that sometimes, lying in that tightly curled never sleeping ball on my bed, I wished for a nail gun to abruptly and violently end it all. The interior of my skull was on fire – I was burning from the inside out and no amount of salty tears could dampen the inferno.

"If you know what's best
Get the Hell away from me."

Tracy Bonham

Unswerving monotony

The two features which dictate time, space and the eternal void in a psychiatric ward are mealtimes and the 'set your watch by' appearance of the medication trolley.

Mealtimes are a crucial cog in the running of the ward as they represent the biggest timewasting event of the day and as such are invaluable to patients. Selecting what to eat is an important ritual too although when it came down to it I actually, in reality, did very little eating during those months.

THE most important thing about mealtimes is unfortunately not revealed to spanking new/terrified to death patients: CHOOSING YOUR SEAT. As such they are left vulnerable to a whole host of social issues. You see, once you pick your seat THAT'S IT – it is totally against protocol to move – I did it once and had to make a round of apologies once I realised my error. Why?

Understandably, the majority of people in that nervous room are dealing with, amongst other things, low self esteem issues and if you intentionally indicate to them that you don't want to sit with them anymore then it's like spitting in their soup! Believe me, it can cause BIG problems. Interestingly, the reason that I moved to a different table in the first place was because I felt paranoid and thought that the people at my table didn't want me there. Go figure!

The medication trolley is the most powerful talisman in the whole place. Alternately, welcomed and resented by the patients (dependent on state of mind), this Aladdin's Cave of psychiatric pharmaceuticals was strictly guarded by at least two nurses when it was wheeled onto the ward. When it was unlocked (with a predictably squeaky key) the lid was lifted and, like a cavernous mouth, displayed a myriad of pills, potions and charts.

Did I ever have a problem with compliancy? Are you kidding? As far as I was concerned if a handful of pills could give me some of this 'sanity' that everyone was talking about then that was fine with me. Pop them in, drink some water, swallow. Done and dusted, thanks very much. How did I feel after taking them? Not much different – a little tired and shaky perhaps but once the doctors and nurses had figured out the right regime for me fairly soon the delusions and hallucinations began to diminish a bit and I began my first tentative steps on the road to recovery. At the very least I could start to sleep again, something I had been deprived of for a good few months, which was a HUGE relief.

"It's a hindrance to my health
If I'm a stranger to myself"

  KT Tunstall

night-and-day-mare

Okay, I didn't have the easiest time when I was ill but even at that point my heart really went out to one patient in the ward who was living a very real but different sort of nightmare to the rest of us. He was a young man, aged around 25, who had been admitted suffering from some kind of psychosis but the more immediate problem was that he was from Iraq and spoke NO ENGLISH!

"Christ!" I remember thinking "What a HORRENDOUS situation to be in! Poor guy." Imagine not being sure, or even worse frightened, of yourself and not being able to speak to someone about it or understand their response. He didn't seem to know what was going on and although we all rallied round there's only so much you can do with gestures and hand signals. The ward staff organised an interpreter but before he arrived the young man tried to smash his bedroom window in with a chair and was transferred to the Intensive Care Unit.

Life is crap sometimes.

PromisesCRUELpromises
(Getting better isn't a straight road)

I was a fish being reeled in, a mug being taken for everything she had in a game of street poker, a drunk promising she could walk a straight line. Mental illness was toying with me, promising sunshine and laughter one day and mocking me with black rain and terrifying screams the next. Getting better, I was to find, does not follow a linear progression. Fits and starts, stits and farts how slowly, so ssssllllloooooowwwwwlllllllllyyyyyyyy things improve then SUDDENLY one afternoon somewhere in between my first and second cup of tea 'click' everything in my brain just locks into place and for the first time in AGES there is silence in my head so much so that I wonder if my ears are blocked with wax.

Tentatively I smile. The World doesn't end. I get up from my seat, find a nurse and gibber "I'm okay, I'm okay! The pills are working – I can go home now!"

I should know better.

All too soon the filthy, trash infested waters, rusty and aching, begin to pour back into the cavities around my pitiful brain contaminating my thoughts and confusing me.

This is the pattern – glimpses of light dashed away like snowflakes melting on an old school radiator – always boiling and cruel. I find myself climbing a ladder and this ladder is scheming: up two rungs, down three – up three, down one. Sores on my hands , splinters in my feet. But you may not stand still so you climb and slip, climb and slip until finally, FINALLY you reach a rung you can bear where the noise is quieted but not gone, the pain is muted but still present and the fear muffled but nagging. You look at the rung above and know it offers better things but you must rest or risk slipping back down. And that scares you more than anything. This ladder has a name and it is a name that becomes clearer with every hard fought passing day: recovery.

"It amazes me — the will of instinct"

Nirvana

Green

Everyone had their own ways of passing time in hospital – some watched mindless daytime TV, some paced the corridors, and others made conversation in the murky smoke room. Me? Well, when I felt well enough I dabbled in all of those activities and the occupational activities on offer in the ward but most of the time I did three things:

1. Lay on my bed with my eyes closed and pretended I didn't exist.

2. Played my guitar

But most of all

3. Watched the trees outside.

More specifically I focused on the leaves and their changing hues dependent on the time of day and weather. It was fascinating and I would spend hours propped up on the safety of my bed staring fixidly out of the window. It's amazing how hugely important details like colour and leaf shape would become to me.

I remember being absolutely FURIOUS at my Mum when she tried to use the trees as a metaphor for my immediate family. NO! They were just my trees, they didn't want personalities nor for that matter need them. Don't fucking bastardize my trees! They were about the only pure thing I had in my life at that point.

I needed them.

Talk to Me

Forget the 'couch'. Forget joyfully leaping to your feet à la Winona Ryder in "Girl Interrupted". Therapy is a hard slog – painful and often humiliating in its revelations. Therapy DEMANDS honesty – to be otherwise wastes everyones' time, especially your own.

I hated it, loved it, resented it, feared it and found, ultimately, that there were no places to hide from it. It was my nemesis. It was my saviour.

Therapy taught me NOT how to beat bipolar but how to accept it and live a 'normal' healthy life with bipolar in tow. Everyday decisions such as should I go to Glasgow for the day, should I buy a CD, should I call a friend for coffee were all made less complex in my head and easier to manage. In the whirling cesspool that was my mind at times, therapy was a calming balm yet one to be careful of as it had teeth. And they were sharp.

"Therapy is Speedie's brand new drug.
Dancing with the Devil's past has never been too fun
It's better off than trying to take a bullet from a gun."

Garbage

them
(more hallucinations)

Insects EVERYWHERE, pursuing me wherever I go. My sticky sheets cling to my legs like malicious cellophane. I open my eyes tentatively, like a child on a sunny morning, and see IT again. Oh, I wish I could describe IT to you but that would just lend IT a reality and solidity that I just can't handle right now. So I'll think of other things as I hide under the pillow. INSECTS. No! INSECTS...... everywhere. Filtering in, dropping by, zoning out. I can feel see, taste, smell and hear them **ALL THE TIME** .

Don't tell me this isn't **REAL**.

Visitors

Receiving visitors in hospital is an odd experience. For one thing you literally count the minutes until they/he/she arrives – constantly checking your watch and increasing the depth of smoke inhalation from your ever waning cigarette supply as the tension mounts. Your ears strain for a familiar tread on the spick and span echoing lino and your eyes flick eagerly over each figure passing the smoke room door.

And then? They ARRIVE! The person(s) who has the sole responsibility of breaking the monotony of your day is here and…and….you have NOTHING TO TALK ABOUT. Like a flaccid balloon they are empty of interest and since all of your days are identical and merge into one the communication barrier between you both is dense, awkward and cringingly embarrassing.

But you need them. They remind you of a life outside and their clothes smell of the rain and travel instead of fag smoke and non scented disinfectant.

"DON'T LEAVE!" you want to scream with every fibre of your being. You rugby tackle them and pin them to the floor craving every moment of companionship. Pity spills from their pores.

"Time to go." Everything says. Suddenly you're so homesick you could cry. So you light another cigarette. They leave. And the clock ticks resolutely on.

Friends

"This place looks like a crematorium!" quipped the male nurse as he entered my room. Mercifully absent of dead bodies I assumed he was referring to the abundance of fragrant flowers which I had been lucky enough to have been sent by friends and family which were littered around the place in impossible-to-cut-yourself-on plastic vases. I was and still am grateful for all of the bouquets I received but my favourites were the two I had been sent by two close Uni friends, Becks and Foye. What made them stand out from the rest? Some rare orchid? Nope. The number of flowers? Uh uh. It was the messages on the cards attached. The one from Becks read "Thinking of you. Take care, love Becks"

Okay, maybe not that unusual but this was immediately followed by Foye's card which hilariously read "BET MY BOUQUET IS BIGGER THAN BECKS'S!!!"

My friends have always known how to make me smile – even when I least expect it!

Scared and analysed

(on a weekly basis)

Once a week, in what was for me a gut wrenching epoch of dread, each inpatient met with the Consultant Psychiatrist. I LOATHED these meetings, or "reviews" as they were known.

I remember the first one in the same way you recall your first bicycle accident – jagged memories awash with shock, numbness and general unpleasantness. I entered the room for my first review unsure of what to expect. What I DIDN'T expect were the eight eager faces that turned to greet me! I was fucking terrified! To understand how frightened I was you have to appreciate that I was having a really hard time summoning up the courage to talk to one person at that point so to be faced with eight was literally paralysing. Suddenly I couldn't speak, swallow or breathe properly. I wanted to leave with every fibre of my being but the door behind me had been closed and anyway, somehow by now I was sitting on a chair beside the Consultant so escape seemed impossible. The Consultant probably asked me some questions about how I was feeling and maybe I even answered – I don't recall. All I know for sure is that there was a slight blue mark on the carpet which struck me as odd since the carpet was brand new. "How strange." I remember thinking. So I stared at it to see if it would burn deeper under my gaze. It didn't.

In the meantime decisions were made about my treatment

that passed like tumbleweed through my dusty brain leaving no mark or trace of their presence. The only comment that carried any resonance at all was when I was told it would be at least a few weeks before the subject of when I would be discharged would be made.

I didn't care. Duvet to hide under. Cigarettes to smoke. Trees to watch. And nurses to keep me safe. That was what I needed at that point and the Ward offered all of those things.

"I'm here but I'm really gone"

Alanis Morissette

Sunday Night Syndrome

Reviews continued to be difficult for me – when you're suffering from depression, delusions and paranoia your perceptions of what people are thinking about you are totally awry and by your thoughts very nature it is impossible to be rational. So I would start to panic on Sunday evening, not sleep on Sunday night, pace and smoke all Monday morning until I was put out of my misery and my name was mercifully called at some point around Monday lunchtime. The reviews themselves were generally short lived affairs which was a huge relief. More than anything I was looking for reassurance from a review – that I was getting better and that I was going to be okay but sometimes I'd be frightened I was going to get sent home to early and at other times that I was going to be kept in for too long.

Reviews continue to be a weekly event in hospital but I think consultants should take the lead from one Psychiatrist who interviews the patient on his own and then reports back to the "masses" thereby causing as little distress to the patient as possible. Makes sense to me!

The System

The manner in which your life was controlled in hospital was entirely dependant on a ratings system. When you were admitted into the somewhat alien yet reassuringly safe confines of the ward you were automatically placed on a '0' which meant an absolute ban on any jaunts outside. Its amazing how quickly you miss the sky, the rain, the feel of the wind in your hair and, of course, it meant you were totally reliant on visitors or other obliging patients for necessities ie. Fanta and fags. (But at least that was better than "special obs" which meant a nurse watching you do EVERYTHING 24 hours a day. Yes, EVERYTHING – shower, pee, brush your teeth, sleep – nothing went unwatched.) Once you had been promoted to a "1" you were allowed out with a nurse accompanying you. Super. I mean the nurses on the ward were cool but everyone needs time to themselves so whilst it was good to be outside I still felt the clawing grip of the hospital on me. A "2", however, was real progress – 15 minutes out on your tod, just enough time to go for a wander, smoke a fag and smile at the local kids pulling "moonies" at you because you were one of those "nutters" they had heard about from their somewhat unenlightened friends. Nice.

When you hit a "3" the walls began to metaphorically fall down around you. You were now allowed out for between half an hour – 1 hour which gave me the luxury of going home, having a coffee, playing with the cat, before heading back over to the ward. I was lucky though, in that we have a car which made the whole process so much easier.

And then, FINALLY, you made it to a "4" (put on the party hats!!!) On this level you are granted pretty much free access outside (after asking permission) and overnight passes of 1, 2, 3 nights in a row are doled out. Should all go well discharge will be just around the corner. All right!

Staying Home

In hospital I floated. There were no external worries other than the relentless noise of my brain. No bills, no stress, no responsibilities then suddenly BAM I was home and faced with EVERYTHING again. I was still fragile and looking at a bill never mind opening and reading it scared the living shit out of me. Luckily my friends and family gathered round, along with my CPN, psychiatrist and GP, to make the transition from being an inpatient to being home again as easy as possible.

I hadn't made myself a meal in a while or driven a car or even bought loo roll so there were huge adjustments to be made. I had to learn to be patient and I'm not a hugely patient person, believe me! Rain surprised me, as did traffic, kids on bikes and pets – after all I had been living in a carefully controlled, artificially safe environment for the past three months. Supermarkets were difficult – too many people too keep an eye on and too much selection. Things I had previously taken for granted or done without thinking had to be planned and prepared for.

But I was home with my family and although I needed sometime to adjust that was a grand place to be and not only that but to start to feel well in myself again. It had been a long journey but I finally felt I was home not only physically but mentally as well. And you know what? I felt a little bit proud of myself and that was something I hadn't felt in a long time. Nice, eh?

"I'm a stranger in this town."

Bush

Part 3 : The Journey Home

Some Thinking Is Getting More Absurd
(Stigma amongst the medical profession)

Look at me. Really look. You're staring at a lucky person. Why? Because even though my life is messed up and confusing as hell at times at least I can voice my worries and concerns. I can go for help. Sure, I've faced stigma – the frightening, paralysing, negative automatic assumptions that the uneducated make about people like me. Like me how? With blond hair? A penchant for blue nail varnish? Nope – those of us who suffer from mental health problems/ challenges/ issues/ (feel free to select one of the above that makes you feel the least uncomfortable). That's what I'm getting at.

It's come glaringly to my attention, however, that there is one surprising group in this supposedly liberal society of ours that is literally terrified of 'coming out' about having a mental illness. And do you know who it is? This may come as a shock – it's our medical profession. The level of stigma in the NHS with regard to mental illness is so prevalent, so absolute, so UNNECESSARY that hundreds, if not thousands, of doctors and countless nurses are struggling to hide their symptoms and cope with the excessive demands of their jobs.

I wrote an article for the British Medical Journal about my 'journey' and received a pile of emails from doctors confiding in me about their own personal struggles. Now coping with mental illness is hard enough but dealing on a daily basis with the very real fear that if you are exposed you stand to lose your career must place an intolerable pressure on that individual. It's not fair and I really hope that in some small way publishing this helps.

So why is there such stigma regarding mental health in the NHS? I believe it ultimately comes down to 3 factors

1. The general unwillingness to go to one's 'peers' when you're mentally in trouble – the worry that somehow you'll be judged as less of a doctor if you admit to struggling with mental health problems of your own and that niggling concern about exactly how confidential are your disclosures when you're speaking to a colleague?

2. Mental illness and all its trappings can't be seen, weighed, or measured and so diagnosis to some people appears vague and uncertain. But, and I swear this on my life, the symptoms that accompany any mental health problem are all too terrifyingly and debilitatingly real.

3. The lack of understanding and yes, fear, of mental illness especially when it affects the medical profession. Doctors are not supposed to get ill. Particularly mentally ill. It implies a type of weakness. Which is the biggest load of bollocks I've heard! Is a doctor with a serious mental illness unfit to work? Ever? Personally, and I realise that this is contentious, I feel that if a medic has a mental health problem but is currently well, taking medication (of course, only if deemed appropriate), seeing a psychiatrist regularly, doing everything to maintain a healthy lifestyle and is willing to listen to others and put his or her hands up and take time out if he or she begins to become ill again then yes, I think it is reasonable to accept that this medic can be part of a supervised team.

But. The fear. Too many people think "mental illness = psycho axe murderer" but literally we are talking about 1 in 4 people will suffer at some time from a mental health problem. There are eight GPs at my local surgery and I'm fine with that.

Doctors and nurses are HUMAN BEINGS and as susceptible to illness, both mental and physical, as the rest of us. I believe this is to everyone's benefit in one important way: empathy. When one person has been 'there' it is easier for them to understand what someone else is going through be it psychosis or chickenpox. Of course, I'm not wishing any sort of illness on anyone but I just find it heartbreaking when I can be treated so superbly in a psychiatric ward and later discover that one nurse had been experiencing difficulties that she was desperately worried would become common knowledge.

I realise that I owe certain doctors and nurses my life – of that I have no doubt – so I find it appalling when 100% of correspondence to me from doctors with mental illness ALL say that they are unable to seek help from their colleagues. That, truly, is a statistic to be both ashamed of and worried by. I thought we lived in a society that was trying to combat all forms of stigma. Maybe I'm naïve. But when the stigma of a condition is so prevalent at the very heart of the Service that is supposed to be treating it?

That more than anything alarms me.

The Mills and Boon bit

I've never really had anyone to miss before. Sure, I miss my family and friends when I'm away from them. But this?? We're talking carve my heart out with a blunt spatula and then stomp all over it with your size 9's. Shit, I miss him. Right now I'm listening to his favourite songs, lying in his bed and pretending he's just popped downstairs to make a cup of tea and that warm, open, good looking but doesn't realise it face will peer round the door and grin at me. But he's not, he's away giving a lecture and the songs make me need him even more and his scent is slowly dissipating from the sheets. Time doesn't heal it just savagely reminds you of what you're missing.

I first met Michel at The Bipolar Fellowship Conference 2005 at King's College, London. Mum and I were due to give a speech but I was feeling absolutely HORRENDOUS for two reasons: 1. I had food poisoning from some extremely dodgy out of date microwave chips which I had unwisely consumed the night before and 2. BECAUSE THERE WERE 300 PEOPLE IN THE AUDIENCE EYEBALLING ME!!! My social phobia was screaming "Where are the exits?" and I was just about to make a run for it when the previous speaker – a rather attractive man in his late forties – wandered over and casually said "Hey, d'ya mind if I sit with you during your talk?" Pretty certain he wasn't/beyond caring if he was a serial killer I gratefully gulped "Yes, please" at which point he gently took the microphone out of my shaking and somewhat embarrassingly sweaty hand and held it firm for me. Then, to cap off the "you are my saviour" routine he whispered phrases such as "good one" "that was great" whenever I opened my mouth and let the words trickle and then eventually pour out.

I spoke to him for about 20 minutes afterwards before being irritatingly swept away to sign books and then, as I had a train to catch, I didn't have another chance to speak to him. However, after some thought and reflection I announced to my Mum as the train pulled into Crewe on the way North that Michel Syrett (I had at least found out his name) was a man I could care for although knowing my luck he was probably married, gay or both! To say that this kind of statement goes against the grain for me is a COLOSSAL understatement – normally I'm a reserved, suss out the situation for a LONG time kind of person. But, and it is impossible not to speak of this without using clichés (hell, it'd be rude not to!) he just seemed like the guy I had been breathing in and out for 33 years for.

So, what did I do next? Call him? Nope. I 'Googled' him (as every 21st Century girl does her potential suitor!). I found out that he was a very accomplished author with around 18 extremely high brow academic text books under his belt. "Shit!" I thought "He must have thought I was a right idiot to be so excited about my poxy wee book. Aaargh!" Mind you, I was hugely impressed that he hadn't played the CV card which would have totally squashed and deflated me. Not a lot of guys would have passed that one up. Nice one Mr Syrett.

Nothing much happened until the following April when I read his column in Pendulum, the Bipolar Fellowship magazine, and was immediately concerned for him. Reading between the lines it was fairly easy to spot that he was struggling mentally and in need of some kind of help. Remembering what he had done for me I decided to answer that call so I emailed him to see if he was okay. He wasn't and was in the middle of a really bad depression. I asked if it would help if I kept the email contact going? He replied that that would be fine although he was feeling pretty low just then. We started emailing, tentatively at first, and then, sooner than either of us had dared hope, Michel's mood began to pick up. Fantastic! That was when the fun began and soon we were emailing up to 30 times a day. It was so EASY – we just never ran out of things to 'talk' about! Nothing like this had ever happened to me before and it continued to defy belief/be pretty nauseating especially when we both sent each other messages that we each thought the other to be our soulmate.......AT THE SAME TIME!!!

Four weeks on and God knows how many crazy, funny, lovely emails later Michel phoned me as he was leaving the country for a few days for works' sake. He left a quick message on my mobile ending with a rather blurted out "I Love you!". Bless him. I emailed him and told him it was reciprocated and with that barrier crossed we decided we needed to meet again to see if there was any chemistry and potential for a regular relationship where we would actually, gasp, SEE each other! Well........one more thing. The evening before Michel was due to meet me he called to say we needed to discuss something. "What HADN'T we discussed?" I replied. "Kids." He said. It turns out that Bipolar runs really strongly in Michel's family and, as he was a bit older, he didn't want kids but felt that if I did we shouldn't meet and he would back off leaving the way clear for me to meet someone who did too. Bless him again. I calmed his fears by reassuring him that I didn't want kids either for the whole Bipolar reason, so not to fret and to get his butt up to Glasgow Central Station, platform 1 ASAP!

The meeting? Me: all sunglasses and trying to look cool. Him: lurking behind other passengers so he could get a good look at me. Finally, after AGES, we spotted each other, awkwardly hugged, kissed and BLOODY-HELL-COR-BLIMEY talk about thunderbolts and lightening!!! We broke apart, stared at each other and said in unison "Oh my God, this is it!"

Dinner followed. I ate nothing – I think I was in shock. I was literally lost for words. All I could do was gulp "this is it!" over and over again whilst we held hands on top of the table.

Looking back I think it was then that he first proposed and I accepted on the condition that I could have a few days to think about it. A girl doesn't like to rush these things. So much was happening so fast, suddenly I was in a Steven Spielberg romantic epic, next we were on the train home (my brother had called to check everything was okay or did I need an escort? I said I was fine.) We were still holding hands and still gazing at each other, trying to cram into my brain as much detail about him as possible. We reached Dalreoch, a nearby station to my hometown, when a young man got on, spotted Michel and myself and uttered the immortal words "Aw, just say 'yes', hen"!!! God, was it that obvious? Apparently so!

Meeting my parents? Hmm. That went kind of well apart from Michel blurting out to my Dad (the kind of man who wears a tie when he gardens) that I was "heat on legs". Aaargh! (Oh yeah, in case you think Michel was just after 'one thing' we actually and genuinely both felt that this relationship had the potential to be SO very special that we held off on intimacy for quite a while so that we could concentrate on romance and getting to know each other first. No big deal, it just turned out to be the right way for both of us.) Back to Dad: mind you, after the nerves (on both sides) had settled and the port was flowing the two of them got on famously. Thank God. Mum had already met Michel at the conference so that was fine and Ollie and he hit it off from the start.

Michel's visit lasted eight wonderful days but don't be fooled, this is the real world and nothing ever goes smoothly. On the third day Michel had an episode of agitated depression which left him confused and wanting to run back to London. He was so miserable, rocking back and forth on my sofa, so I hugged him and we talked. Finally I put him to bed as he was exhausted but we had made it through that little crisis and that was to stand us in good stead as a couple. When he woke I played him a song that we both identified with, Alanis Morissette's "Everything" – I love his light and dark too.

On the fourth day when things were much brighter and breezier Michel announced that we had a major problem.

Geography. After all, he lived in London which made things difficult to say the least. Then he said something so giving and unselfish that I got goose pimples. He said he couldn't take me away from my hometown as it was obvious that I had major roots there but how would I feel if he, and his 84 year old Mum, whom he visited daily moved, and bought a house up here? I was blown away. No one had ever even vaguely offered to do something like that for me. He was and is a truly amazing man.

So here we are, some 14 very stressful months later with Michel and his mum now firmly ensconsed in a lovely Edwardian house just round from my flat. Moving is well known as being one of the most stressful events anyone can go through and this one was not to be without its moments either - with some unexpected difficulties and crises - but all these additional stresses and strains only succeeded in bringing us closer together. I love him with everything I have and have yet to acquire. Yes, we will marry but we'll wait and see when it feels right. No meringues though!

And to think that both of us nearly pulled out of that conference, me because I wasn't well and him because of jet lag. It's not for me to decide for you whether you believe in God or even fate; all I'm saying is that someone was definitely watching that day.

And my cat LOVES him!

*"You see all my light and you love my dark
.........And you're still here."*

Alanis Morissette

What Do You Do?

How comfortable am I about the fact that I take psychiatric medication three times a day? Pretty comfortable, actually. Why? The answer is twofold: firstly I believe that it helps me cope with the condition I have and secondly because I believe we all have the right to choose and be respected for the choices that we make in life, at least with regard to whether we take medication or not. So just because I take medication doesn't mean I'm going to get all preachy to those who choose other forms of treatment. I hope I'm not asking too much to say that I hope for the same respect in return.

Mental illness is tough enough without forgetting that it is the symptoms we are supposed to be battling and not each others ideas and viewpoints. If whatever you're doing works for you (and it's not illegal or harming anyone else) then keep doing it.

Whatever, the situation, it takes many different coping mechanisms to manage mental illness or whatever. Just remember that we are all different and what works for one might not necessarily work for another.

TURN UP THAT VOLUME CONTROL!!!

Music impacts more on our lives nowadays than it did at any time during history. It is pretty much impossible to escape (should we want to) and the diversity of styles available to us is breathtaking – jazz to classical, rock to dance, hip hop to world and many, many more – we are a veritable ocean of textures, sounds, dynamics and beats.

Adverts use music to court our fancies, TV programmes to enhance their message; be it punchline or climax and of course there is the colossal music industry which runs itself ragged trying both to dictate and predict what we will/won't/just might like and so download or buy to appease that nagging urge in our brains that tells us that we MUST own that particular piece of music. Why? Hmmm.....good question. Now before we open a philosophical NIGHTMARE and ask "But why do we like/need ANYTHING?" let's hold our horses and remember it's MUSIC that we're talking about here. That's all. Hang on a minute – THAT'S ALL???!!!!!!!

Music, or at least certain genres of it, run a close second to food and water in some peoples' book (mine included). The aural stimulation, reassurance and feeling that I am not alone in my angst has helped me through many difficult times when I have been well and truly in the vicious grip of bipolar and psychosis. Not only do I listen to music I write and perform my own something I find therapeutic not only for myself but hopefully for others as my band's (Bad Alice) music is all about mental illness and social issues that affect young people.

I think I'll always consider myself musically naïve. Sure, if you ask me about any American band during '91-'94 I could probably do a "Mastermind" spot on that particular era but I'm embarrassed at my ignorance of jazz or classical music, for that matter. I love punk, emo, grunge, rock, blues, acoustic but that doesn't and shouldn't stop me from wanting to be open to other forms of music and welcoming their potentially helpful and psychologically soothing effects onto my CD player.

The reason I learnt to play music (the guitar) is steeped in mental illness. I dropped out of Uni because of bipolar, bought a extraordinarily cheap guitar off a friend for £5 and found, to my huge relief and delight, that if I spent time teaching myself to play the 'bad thoughts' and depressive loomings would recede. I needed no encouragement to practice! When I was admitted to hospital they let me take my guitar with me and my "music therapy" as such became a huge part of my road to recovery.

Sure, not everyone's musical, but try even keeping a beat with your foot when listening to something. It might just help.

A World of Difference

*(My ideal description of a place of treatment
should I become ill again)*

Silence. And leaves in the sunshine. No unpredictable barking dogs or lurchings on a train. Everything calm and secure. Sanctuary. Asylum, in the best and truest sense of the word. Not to be torn away and processed but nurtured and embraced. Space for all of those who need. Clean, comfortable, supported, *safe*. Not cold, hungry or lonely. Not alienated, confused, scared and intimidated by unknown surroundings or strangers. No pressure. Just time. And healing.

How do we begin?

How do we sustain?

How do we succeed?

Needed

(One of the biggest triggers of mental illness
is lack of sleep)

I stalk you, tapping your unsuspecting yet inherently weary shoulder. You try to run from me, to deny me but I am everywhere – waiting and not to be feared. I am your best friend. I am your blanket when you were three years old. I contain all your dreams. I hold all your nightmares. Without me you will wither and fade like a flower hidden from the sun. I WILL have your attention and the more you welcome me the more you gain. Lose me and therein lies the trigger for untold carnage both mentally and physically.

Come to me and lay down in my arms.

For I am Sleep.

razor wire corset

(Stress, and what it does to you!)

If all the pages in this book were blank it would still not even begin to reflect the vacant lurchings of my mind at this current moment. Stress stalks me like a feral cat and I feel cold and seasick on an ocean of truculent sand that rubs my insides bloody and raw.

The invisible barbed, no, RAZOR wire corset returns and, with every faltering breath, mercilessly binds tighter and tighter around my abdomen. Pop a sturdy stick into the mix and an insane tourniquet of fresh pain and torment merrily begins. Who, What, Where is to blame? The answer is the only clear thing I have. Me. To the World nothing shows (I have been oh so careful about this) but inside? I rot and rust, clank and grind, like an unoiled chain on an aging uncared for bicycle. How I hate this.

Slimy antacids rule my world and if I were to vomit it would be red as my guts told their piteous stories in a heady mixture of bile and blood.

Eating has become a Purgatory state – will it hurt? Won't it? I eye even a sympathetic banana as it turns into jagged steel in accordance with one of those false teeth adverts. Milk? Milk is nectar and I swig on various varieties all day. And my Beloved? My Beloved takes pity on me, pops round and lowers his mighty cooking skills to macaroni cheese.

"I'd walk a thousand miles to slip this skin"

Bruce Springsteen

Hello......?

Hey babe, you sleeping? I need you RIGHT NOW 'cos it's dark and I'm barely hanging on here with my ragged, chewed and bleeding fingernails. I'm scared, babe, and I think if you were to envelop me in the warmth of your arms it...might...just...help.

I'm a cat in a bag with a brick and wicked intentions looming, I'm a rabbit in the hungry sights of a gun and I'm a fresh, green lawn about to be mown.

Wake up,babe........

I'll whisper my distress 'cos you look so peaceful. I can see tomorrow's stubble peeking through your chin and only we know that in a few long hours it'll be spinning away down the plughole.

Wake up, babe. I need you, I love you, I can't live... no wait, there was something more I think, not sure now.

Help me, babe, turnaround these grating thoughts in my weary brain and let me sleep a sleep sent from Heaven – filled with dreams of me and you.

I'm dying here, babe. Slowly. And I seem to be the only one who is around to watch and listen.

...It isn't really that much of a show........

Wake up, babe (please).   Wake up.

bond

I found him in the sitting room at 2am, lying curled up in the foetal position, all alone in the dark rhythmically hitting his head off the wooden floor. His eyes were shut and he was freezing cold – I'd only just woken up so God knows how long he'd been there. I called his name. No response. I went to hug him. He was rigid

What do you DO in these circumstances? How do you get the ball rolling forwards again? You get practical. There is no time for tears. They can come later. First a cushion under his head, then a duvet to warm him up, followed by a call to the emergency doctor on my mobile so that I don't have to leave him for longer than necessary, finally just crawling under the duvet, holding him tight and waiting , praying, hoping that everything will be okay.

You talk to him continuously about how much you love him and, after an hour, he opens his eyes and then, after two, he sits up. You help him drink a half filled sweetened cup of tea because he's shaking so much you can hear his teeth chatter. And then the doctor arrives and, holding your boyfriend's hand, you try really hard to remember everything that has happened and report it in an unemotional 'no that didn't rip me apart' fashion. The doctor leaves some medicine and you both go to bed to try and sleep and see what tomorrow brings.

This is what it is like from the other side. This is what it is like for so many couples including Michel and myself who both suffer from a mental illness. But there is more, so much more. There is the implicit understanding that we both need our meds and must get enough sleep. We understand and empathise with how the symptoms of our own particular illnesses affect us. He'll remind me to take my pills in the morning and I'll tell him when he should think about going to see the doctor. Quid pro quo. It works. It really does. However, we are two people who are educated in our illnesses and are aware of the pitfalls and the boobytraps that surround them – those triggers or personal incidents that can cause our mental health to lurch into a dramatic downward spiral. Sure, we still get ill but we are both constantly vigilant for both our own and each others warning signs that things might be about to go awry.

However, let's face it, I'm not in this relationship to protect either of our conditions (although of course we do). I'm in it because I've found the man who can make me, in turn, laugh, love, dream, hope and lie on a freezing wooden floor at 2am for three hours without causing me a seconds' complaint.

A day like any other

Play table tennis with a large Fresian. Open eyes. Realise I was dreaming. Look at Michel. God, I'm lucky. Turn on stereo. Garbage asks "Why do you love me?". Get up. Trip over slippers. Make tea. Consider killing myself. Go upstairs. Have breakfast with Michel. Shower. Eject wet, yelling cat from bathroom. No bloody soap left. Dry off. Put on selection of clothes. Snog Michel. Hmm. Snog Michel again. Look out of the window. Sunshine and early risers. Seagulls soar. Long drop to the pavement below. Put dirty clothes in washing machine. Remove cat from washing machine. Take medication. Change cat litter, feed and water cat. Leave house with Michel. Drive to Tesco's. Buy paper and fruit juice. Say "Hi" to Trisha who serves me. Drive to parents. Wait for Michel. Drink fruit juice and check emails. Michel arrives and starts work. Want my life to stop. Laugh at a joke. Play my guitar. Read the paper. Start a new chapter in book. Inspiration required. Not forthcoming. Bugger. Hug Michel. Eat two boiled eggs for lunch (okay, and some cocopops – sod the diet). Take medication. Catch forty winks with Michel. We tell each other secrets of how much we love each other. Get up. Look in mirror. Creased face and hair sticking up at weird angles. Ah well. Transcribe more of book. Eat some chicken bites. Play guitar. Desperate suicidal thoughts. Pick up Ollie from the station. Michel finishes work. Say "bye" to Mum. Go to pub for a coffee. Head to Michel's house. Chat to his Mum. Eat dinner cooked by Michel.

Cuddle. Watch 'Green Wing'. Take medication. Kiss Michel and tell him to sleep tight. Roll onto right side with right foot sticking out of duvet. Close eyes. Return to the land of table tennis playing cows.

Coping Strategies

I'm still here. And therein lies my message. Mental illness can destroy, distract, disable and cause untold damage to the sufferer and those around him/her but there are methods and techniques that I employ to ease the pain and speed up my recovery. These are simple plans of action that help me live a more positive life and if you feel that they might offer you some assistance feel free to use them. A degree in rocket science is not required.

1. Go and see your GP *when you are well* and explain what your 'warning signs' are. By this I mean the early changes in mood, behaviour or thought patterns that ring your alarm bells. By disclosing this to your GP you will find that you are both better able to gauge when you need help and early intervention means that you are less likely to experience a full blown episode.

2. Buy some small notebooks and fill them with information about your condition ie the medication that you are taking (if any), questions to ask you if you are ill (Do you feel like harming yourself, Are you having any scary thoughts etc.), emergency phone numbers, a description of you symptoms.

   Once you have completed them give them to the people you are around the most so that they will be more likely to spot if you are becoming unwell and act accordingly.

3. Eat as healthily as you can and avoid alcohol. Alcohol is a major depressant and can stop medication from working effectively.

4. Do not do illegal drugs.

5. Try and go for a long walk every day or, if the weather's crap, try and get some form of exercise.

6. If you're unwell and you don't feel like talking to friends or family phone a registered helpline like Samaritans, Saneline or Breathing Space. Sometimes it can be easier talking to a trained, non judgemental stranger and remember two things: you are NOT wasting their time and you can hang up when you feel like it.

7. Give yourself at least one thing to look forward to everyday. For example, go round to a friend's house for coffee, or, if you can afford it, buy a magazine. Visit the nearest library – it's free and it's warm and you can even read! I tend to play my guitar or visit a friend. Find out what works for you and enjoy it.

8. Get loads of sleep.

9. I find feeling and sniffing an orange or grapefruit very helpful and helps to distract me from my thoughts.

10. Never give up on yourself. You're too important.

Finally (a new beginning)

Some things are meant to happen to us. So are others. As I mentioned earlier, it's like a hand of cards that we are dealt and, regardless of whether you have a mental illness or not, its how you play those cards that determines how your life turns out. My life is turning out okay. Yes, I am still troubled by truly awful thoughts and moods but I am able to equally recognise the good in my life and I hope I embrace it.

Most of the things that I wrote about in this book happened several years ago but I felt it was important to remove their dusty sleeves and give them a spin on my laptop once again. The reason for this? I felt that enough time had passed for me to truly reflect on and be open about the horrors and nightmares that had tortured me daily. I am all too readily aware that that I am not alone in having these terrifying, all consuming thoughts and feelings. I wanted to put 'pen to paper' to give recognition to those demons so that others, like me, can identify and assuage what is going on in their heads.

This is my hope. This is my purpose. Only you can judge if it was my success.

> "When the day is long
> And the night,
> The night is yours alone.
> When you think you've had
> Too much of this life,
> Hold on."
>
> R.E.M

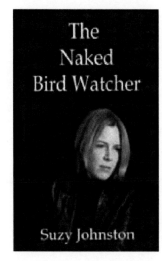

The Naked Bird Watcher

ISBN 0954809203

Too often writers approach mental illness from the outside; this is one of the rare books which puts you in the shoes of the person experiencing mental distress. Suzy literally takes you along in the terrifying descent into the dark, murky world of mental illness in which she found herself, unaware and unprepared for what was happening to her. With vivid descriptions, you join her as she realizes 'that something, somehow was horribly wrong'. You are there as she suffers the apathy ad dullness her life is becoming, too paralyzed to care. In what otherwise would be a typical collegiate experience: meeting new friends, partying late into the night, competing with the Hockey Club, learning guitar and joining a local band.....Suzy faced the added confusion of dealing with an insidious illness which was slowly turning her life inside out, yet elusively escaped being pinned down and understood. She writes of experiences with doctors unsure or unable to give a diagnosis and hospitalisation. You experience her initial fear of hospital admission yet you also experience the first steps on the road to her recovery. Overall, the care she received was excellent and really established the fundamental steps for her on-going recovery and provided her with the tools to cope and manage the symptoms of her condition. She learned to recognise the signs that she needs help and how to get it. This positive aspect of her account is one of the true strengths of the book. There is a model for success here which many can learn from, yet there is still valuable constructive suggestions which come from her own experience.

The book is an easy read and one you will not forget. It will give you a new degree of compassion, respect and understanding for the brave souls who deal with mental illness. Her honest and moving account of her struggles and progress serves as an inspiration to the rest of us and will undoubtedly help many who suffer from the devastating symptoms of mental illness as well as those who love and help them when they need it.

Suzy Johnston writes in an easy style with good humour and an incredible ability to both convey her innermost feelings in these experiences and an impartial view of what happened to her – it is that unique ability that sets her and her writing apart.

Doug Huskey NAMI, USA

Available from all bookshops, internet bookstores and www.thecairn.com

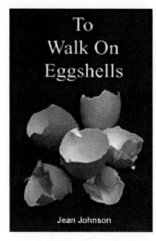

Jean Johnson

To Walk on Eggshells

ISBN 0954809211

This is a priceless account of the agony, shock, love and stamina of a mother faced with a child who has been dealt the unkind hand of severe mental illness. Easy to read, clearly sincere and uncontrived it is altogether memorable. Her feelings are described with endearing honesty and simplicity, over the space of several years and through the various stages of her daughter's illness and recovery. Her early feelings of utter uselessness are so real and understandable, the only solace coming from basic mothering activities such as ironing her daughter's pyjamas on the eve of being admitted to a psychiatric unit.

One of the many remarkable features of this account is Jean's appreciation of the irreplaceable role of in-patient care, when sanctuary is needed, and the oft repeated affection for specialist staff. She bucks the fashionable trend of demanding a right to be involved in the detail of her daughter's hospital care, recognising the dangers of over involvement and seeing her daughter's relationship with her teams as her own business. Her relationship with the ward cleaner is a great comfort and is a useful reminder of the totality of a service which is discounted by planners and managers.

Altogether this is a refreshingly sensible and emotionally

riveting account from an intelligent lady who is blessed with the unusual combination of modesty, insight and the energetic desire to do something to ease the plight of those afflicted with mental illness.

Professor AVP Mackay, OBE, MA, BSc (Pharm), PhD, MB, ChB, FRCP (Ed), FRCPsych, Tpsych, Director of Mental Health Services, Lomond and Argyll (retired)

Available from all bookshops, internet bookstores and www.thecairn.com

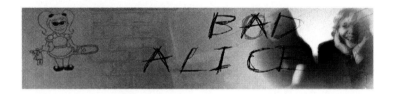

'Mental illness is what I have – not who I am'

Suzy Johnston, August 2007

Bad Alice music highlights a reflective yet positive message on coping with mental distress, self-harm and comments on the challenges and social pressures that face the youth of today.

The Bad Alice CD 'Walk in my Shoes' is available at Bookworms, Helensburgh – purchase or download from www.badalicemusic.com

Lightning Source UK Ltd.
Milton Keynes UK
06 May 2010

153759UK00001B/105/P